THE DASH DIET COOKBOOK

Ultimate Handbook to Cook with Low Sodium Recipes.

Lower your Blood Pressure with Quick, Simple and Easy Delicious Meals to Eat Everyday for Hypertension.

Alexangel Kitchen

Just for Our Readers

To Thank You for Purchasing the Book, for a limited time, you can get a Special FREE BOOK from Alexangel Kitchen

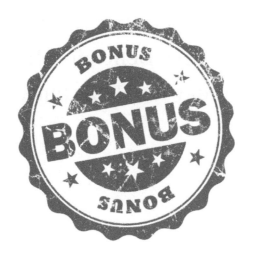

Just go to
https://alexangelkitchen.com/ to
download your FREE BOOK

Table of Contents

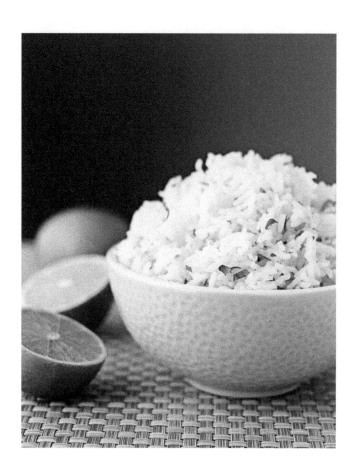

Vegetable Cheese Calzone

Preparation time: 15 minutes

Cooking time: 20 minutes

Servings: 4

Ingredients:

- 3 asparagus stalks, cut into pieces

- 1/2 cup spinach, chopped

- 1/2 cup broccoli, chopped

- 1/2 cup sliced

- 2 tablespoons garlic, minced

- 2 teaspoons olive oil, divided

- 1/2 lb. frozen whole-wheat bread dough, thawed

- 1 medium tomato, sliced

- 1/2 cup mozzarella, shredded

- 2/3 cup pizza sauce

Directions:

1. Prepare the oven to 400 degrees F to preheat. Grease a baking sheet with cooking oil and set it aside. Toss asparagus with mushrooms, garlic, broccoli, and spinach in a bowl. Stir in 1 teaspoon

---

olive oil and mix well. Heat a greased skillet on medium heat.

2. Stir in vegetable mixture and sauté for 5 minutes. Set these vegetables aside. Cut the bread dough into quarters.

3. Spread each bread quarter on a floured surface into an oval. Add sautéed vegetables, 2 tbsp cheese, and tomato slice to half of each oval.

4. Wet the edges of each oval and fold the dough over the vegetable filling. Pinch and press the two edges.

5. Place these calzones on the baking sheet. Brush each calzone with foil and bake for 10 minutes. Heat pizza sauce in a saucepan for a minute. Serve the calzone with pizza sauce.

Nutritional:

Calories 198

Fat 8 g

Sodium 124 mg

Carbs 36 g

Protein 12 g

Mixed Vegetarian Chili

Preparation time: 10 minutes

Cooking time: 36 minutes

Servings: 4

Ingredients:

- 1 tablespoon olive oil

- 14 oz. canned black beans, rinsed and drained

- ½ cup yellow Onion, chopped

- 12 oz. extra-firm tofu, cut into pieces

- 14 oz. canned kidney beans, rinsed and drained

- 2 cans (14 oz.) diced tomatoes

- 3 tablespoons chili powder

- 1 tablespoon oregano

- 1 tablespoon chopped cilantro (fresh coriander)

Directions:

1. Take a soup pot and heat olive oil in it over medium heat. Add onions and sauté for 6 minutes until soft. Add tomatoes, beans, chili powder, oregano, and beans. Boil it first, then reduce the heat to a simmer. Cook for 30 minutes, then add cilantro. Serve warm.

Nutrition:

Calories 314

Fat 6 g

Sodium 119 mg

Carbs 46g

Protein 19 g

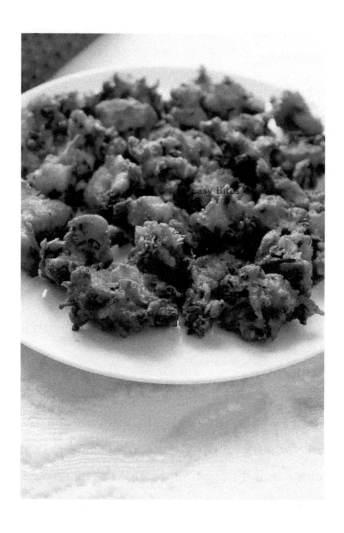

Zucchini Pepper Kebabs

Preparation time: 15 minutes

Cooking time: 40 minutes

Servings: 2

Ingredients:

- 1 small zucchini, sliced into 8 pieces

- 1 red onion, cut into 4 wedges

- 1 green bell pepper, cut into 4 chunks

- 8 cherry tomatoes

- 8 button mushrooms

- 1 red bell pepper, cut into 4 chunks

- 1/2 cup Italian dressing, fat-free

- 1/2 cup brown rice

- 1 cup of water

- 4 wooden skewers, soaked and drained

Directions:

1. Toss tomatoes with zucchini, onion, peppers, and mushrooms in a bowl. Stir in Italian dressing and mix well to coat the vegetables. Marinate them for 10 minutes. Boil water with rice in a saucepan, then reduce the heat to a simmer.

2. Cover the rice and cook for 30 minutes until rice is done. Meanwhile, prepare the grill and preheat it on medium heat. Grease the grilling rack with cooking spray and place it 4 inches above the heat.

3. Thread 2 mushrooms, 2 tomatoes, and 2 zucchini slices along with 1 onions wedge, 1 green and red pepper slice on each skewer. Grill these kebabs for 5 minutes per side. Serve warm with boiled rice.

Nutrition:

Calories 335

Fat 8.2 g

Sodium 516 mg

Carbs 67 g

Protein 8.8 g

Asparagus Cheese Vermicelli

Preparation time: 10 minutes

Cooking time: 15 minutes

Servings: 4

Ingredients:

- 2 teaspoons olive oil, divided

- 6 asparagus spears, cut into pieces

- 4 oz. dried whole-grain vermicelli

- 1 medium tomato, chopped

- 1 tablespoon garlic, minced

- 2 tablespoons fresh basil, chopped

- 4 tablespoons Parmesan, freshly grated, divided

- 1/8 teaspoon black pepper, ground

Directions:

1. Add 1 tsp oil to a skillet and heat it. Stir in asparagus and sauté until golden brown.

2. Cut the sautéed asparagus into 1-inch pieces. Fill a sauce pot with water up to ¾ full. After boiling the water, add pasta and cook for 10 minutes until it is all done.

3. Drain and rinse the pasta under tap water. Add pasta to a large bowl, then toss in olive oil, tomato, garlic, asparagus, basil, garlic, and parmesan. Serve with black pepper on top.

Nutrition:

Calories 325

Fat 8 g

Sodium 350 mg

Carbs 48 g

Protein 7.3 g

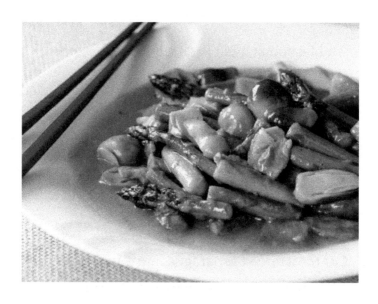

Corn Stuffed Peppers

Preparation time: 10 minutes

Cooking time: 35 minutes

Servings: 4

Ingredients:

- 4 red or green bell peppers

- 1 tablespoon olive oil

- ¼ cup onion, chopped

- 1 green bell pepper, chopped

- 2 1/2 cups fresh corn kernels

- 1/8 teaspoon chili powder

- 2 tablespoons chopped fresh parsley

- 3 egg whites

- 1/2 cup skim milk

- 1/2 cup water

Directions:

1. Prepare the oven to 350 F to preheat. Layer a baking dish with cooking spray. Cut the bell peppers from the top and remove their seeds from inside. Put the peppers in your prepared baking dish with their cut side up.

2. Add oil to a skillet, then heat it on medium flame. Stir in onion, corn, and green pepper. Sauté for 5 minutes. Add cilantro and chili powder. Switch the heat to low. Mix milk plus egg whites in a bowl. Pour this mixture into the skillet and cook for 5 minutes while stirring.

3. Divide this mixture into each pepper. Add some water to the baking dish. Cover the stuffed peppers with an aluminum sheet. Bake for 15 minutes, then serves warm.

Nutrition:

Calories 197

Fat 5 g

Sodium 749 mg

Carbs 29 g

Protein 9 g

Stuffed Eggplant Shells

Preparation time: 10 minutes

Cooking time: 25 minutes

Servings: 2

Ingredients:

- 1 medium eggplant

- 1 cup of water

- 1 tablespoon olive oil

- 4 oz. cooked white beans

- 1/4 cup onion, chopped

- 1/2 cup red, green, or yellow bell peppers, chopped

- 1 cup canned unsalted tomatoes

- 1/4 cup tomatoes liquid

- 1/4 cup celery, chopped

- 1 cup fresh mushrooms, sliced

- 3/4 cup whole-wheat breadcrumbs

- Freshly ground black pepper, to taste

Directions:

1. Prepare the oven to 350 degrees F to preheat. Grease a baking dish with cooking spray and set it

aside. Trim and cut the eggplant into half, lengthwise. Scoop out the pulp using a spoon and leave the shell about ¼ inch thick.

2. Place the shells in the baking dish with their cut side up. Add water to the bottom of the dish. Dice the eggplant pulp into cubes and set them aside. Add oil to an iron skillet and heat it over medium heat. Stir in onions, peppers, chopped eggplant, tomatoes, celery, mushrooms, and tomato juice.

3. Cook for 10 minutes on simmering heat, then stirs in beans, black pepper, and breadcrumbs. Divide this mixture into the eggplant shells. Cover the shells with a foil sheet and bake for 15 minutes. Serve warm.

Nutrition:

Calories 334

Fat 10 g

Sodium 142 mg

Carbs 35 g

Protein 26 g

Southwestern Vegetables Tacos

Preparation time: 10 minutes

Cooking time: 20 minutes

Servings: 4

Ingredients:

- 1 tablespoon olive oil

- 1 cup red onion, chopped

- 1 cup yellow summer squash, diced

- 1 cup green zucchini, diced

- 3 large garlic cloves, minced

- 4 medium tomatoes, seeded and chopped

- 1 jalapeno chili, seeded and chopped

- 1 cup fresh corn kernels

- 1 cup canned pinto, rinsed and drained

- 1/2 cup fresh cilantro, chopped

- 8 corn tortillas

- 1/2 cup smoke-flavored salsa

Directions:

1. Add olive oil to a saucepan, then heat it over medium heat. Stir in onion and sauté until soft. Add zucchini and summer squash. Cook for 5 minutes.

2. Stir in corn kernels, jalapeno, garlic, beans, and tomatoes. Cook for another 5 minutes. Stir in cilantro, then remove the pan from the heat.

3. Warm each tortilla in a dry nonstick skillet for 20 secs per side. Place the tortilla on the serving plate. Spoon the vegetable mixture in each tortilla. Top the mixture with salsa. Serve.

Nutrition:

Calories 310

Fat 6 g

Sodium 97 mg

Carbs 54 g

Protein 10g

Soups

Chicken and Tortilla Soup

Preparation time: 15 minutes

Cooking time: 6 hours

Servings: 12

Ingredients:

- 3 Chicken Breasts (boneless and skinless)

- 15 ounces diced Tomatoes

- 10 ounces Enchilada Sauce

- 1 chopped onion (med.)

- 4 ounces chopped Chili Pepper (green)

- 3 minced cloves Garlic

- 2 cups Water

- 14.5-ounces Chicken Broth (fat-free)

- 1 tbsp. Cumin

- 1 tbs. Chile Powder

- 1 tsp. Salt

- ¼ tsp. Black Pepper

- Bay Leaf

- 1 tbsp. Cilantro (chopped)

- 10 ounces Frozen Corn

- 3 tortillas, cut into thin slices

Directions:

1. Put all the listed fixing in the slow cooker. Stir well to mix. Cook on low heat within 8 hrs. or high heat for 6 hrs. Shred the chicken breasts to a plate. Add chicken to other ingredients. Serve hot, garnished with tortilla slices.

Nutrition:

Calories 93.4

Fat 1.9 g

Cholesterol 18.6

Sodium 841.3 mg

Carbohydrates 11.9 g

Fiber 2.1 g

Protein 8.3 g

Stuffed Pepper Soup

Preparation time: 15 minutes

Cooking time: 8 hours & 10 minutes

Servings: 6

Ingredients:

- 1 lb. ground Beef (drained)

- 1 chopped onion (large)

- 2 cups Tomatoes (diced)

- 2 chopped Green Peppers

- 2 cups Tomato Sauce

- 1 tbs. Beef Bouillon

- 3 cups of water

- Pepper

- 1 tsp. of Salt

- 1 cup of cooked rice (white)

Directions:

1. Place all ingredients in a cooker. Cook for 8 hours on "low." Serve hot.

Nutrition:

Calories 216.1

Fat 5.1 g

Cholesterol 43.4 mg

Sodium 480.7 mg

Carbohydrates 21.8 mg

Fiber 2.5 g

Protein 18.8 g

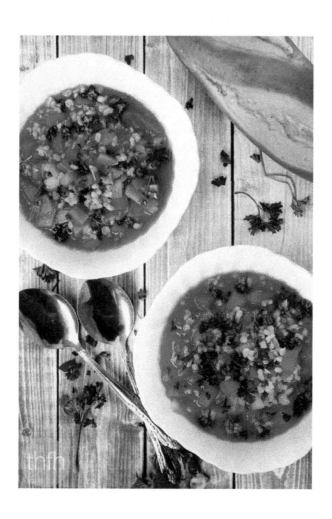

Ham and Pea Soup

Preparation time: 15 minutes

Cooking time: 8 hours

Servings: 8

Ingredients:

- 1 lb. Split Peas (dried)

- 1 cup sliced Celery

- 1 cup sliced Carrots

- 1 cup sliced Onion

- 2 cups chopped ham (cooked)

- 8 cups of water

Directions:

1. Place all the listed fixing in the slow cooker. Cook on "high" within 4 hrs. Serve hot.

Nutrition:

- Calories 118.6

- Fat 1.9 g

- Cholesterol 15.9 mg

- Sodium 828.2 mg

- Carbohydrates 14.5 mg

- Fiber 5.1 g

- Protein 11.1 g

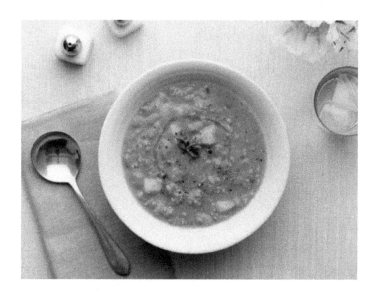

Pea Soup

Preparation time: 15 minutes

Cooking time: 8 hours

Servings: 8

Ingredients:

- 16 oz. Split Peas (dried)

- 1 cup chopped Baby Carrots

- 1chopped onion (white)

- 3 Bay Leaves

- 10 oz. cubed Turkey Ham

- 4 cubes Chicken Bouillon

- 7 cups of water

Directions:

1. Rinse and drain peas. Place all the fixing in the slow cooker. Cook on "low" for 8 hrs. Serve hot.

Nutrition:

Calories 122.7

Fat 2 g

Cholesterol 24 mg

Sodium 780.6 mg

Carbohydrates 15 mg

Fiber 5.2 g

Protein 11.8 g

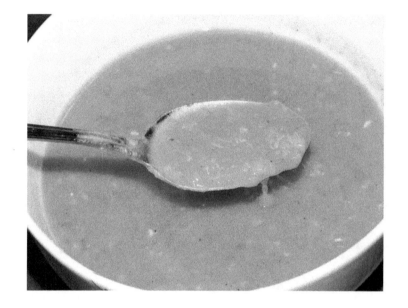

Soup for The Day

Preparation time: 15 minutes

Cooking time: 10 hours & 10 minutes

Servings: 8

Ingredients:

- 1 Beef Steak (cubed)

- 1 chopped onion (med.)

- 1 tbsp. Olive Oil

- 5 thinly sliced med. Carrots

- 4 cups Cabbage

- 4 diced Red Potatoes

- 2 diced Celery Stalks

- 2 cans Tomatoes, diced

- 2 cans Beef Broth

- 1 tsp. Sugar

- 1 can Tomato Soup

- 1 tsp. Parsley Flakes (dried)

- 2 tsp. Italian Seasoning

Directions:

1. In a skillet, sauté onion, and steak in oil. Transfer the sautéed mixture to the slow cooker. Put the rest of the fixing in the slow cooker. Cook on "low" for 10 hrs. Serve hot.

Nutrition:

Calories 259.6

Fat 6.7 g

Cholesterol 29.8 mg

Sodium 699.2 mg

Carbohydrates 31.6 mg

Fiber 4.6 g

Protein 18.9 g

Chipotle Squash Soup

Preparation time: 15 minutes

Cooking time: 4 hours & 20 minutes

Servings: 6

Ingredients:

- 6 cups Butternut Squash (cubed)

- ½ cup chopped Onion

- 2 tsp. Adobo Chipotle

- 2 cups Chicken Broth

- 1 tbsp. Brown Sugar

- ¼ cup Tart Apple (chopped)

- 1 cup Yogurt (Greek style)

- 2 tbsp. Chives (chopped)

Directions:

1. Except for yogurt, chives, and apple, place all the ingredients in the slow cooker. Cook on "low" for 4 hrs. Now, in a blender or food processer, puree the cooked ingredients. Transfer puree to slow cooker.

2. Put the yogurt and cook on "Low" within 20 more mins. Garnish with chives and apples. Serve hot in heated bowls.

Nutrition:

Calories 102

Fat 11 g

Cholesterol 2 mg

Sodium 142 mg

Carbohydrates 22 mg

Fiber 3 g

Protein 4 g

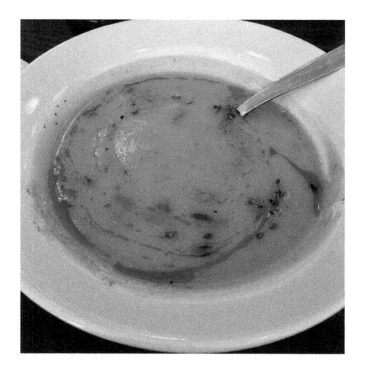

Kale Verde

Preparation time: 15 minutes

Cooking time: 6 hours

Servings: 6

Ingredients:

- ¼ cup Olive Oil (extra virgin)

- 1 Yellow Onion (large)

- 2 cloves Garlic

- 2 ounces Tomatoes, dried

- 2 cups Yellow Potatoes (diced)

- 14-ounce Tomatoes (diced)

- 6 cups Chicken broth

- White pepper (ground)

- 1-pound o chopped Kale

Directions:

1. Sauté onion for 5 mins in oil. Add the garlic and sauté again for 1 minute. Transfer the sautéed mixture to the slow cooker. Put the rest of the fixing except pepper into the slow cooker. Cook on "low" for 6 hrs. Season with white pepper to taste. Serve hot in heated bowls

---

Nutrition:

Calories 257

Fat 22 g

Cholesterol 3 mg

Sodium 239 mg

Carbohydrates 27 mg

Fiber 6 g

Protein 14 g

Escarole with Bean Soup

Preparation time: 15 minutes

Cooking time: 6 hours

Servings: 6

Ingredients:

- 1 tbsp. Olive Oil

- 8 crushed cloves Garlic

- 1 cup chopped Onions

- 1 diced Carrot

- 3 tsp. Basil (dried)

- 3 tsp. Oregano (dried)

- 4 cups Chicken Broth

- 3 cups chopped Escarole

- 1 cup of Northern Beans (dried)

- Parmesan Cheese (grated)

- 14 ounces o Tomatoes (diced)

Directions:

1. Sauté garlic for 2 mins in oil using a large soup pot. Except for the cheese, broth, and beans, add the rest of the ingredients and cook for 5 mins. Transfer the cooked ingredients to the slow cooker.

2. Mix in the broth and beans. Cook on "low" for 6 hrs. Garnish with cheese. Serve hot in heated bowls.

Nutrition:

Calories 98

Fat 33 g

Cholesterol 1 mg

Sodium 115 mg

Carbohydrates 14 mg

Fiber 3 g

Protein 8 g

Chicken Squash Soup

Preparation time: 15 minutes

Cooking time: 5 hours & 30 minutes

Servings: 3

Ingredients:

- ½ Butternut Squash (large)

- 1 clove Garlic

- 1 ¼ quarts broth (vegetable or chicken)

- 1/8 tsp. Pepper (white)

- ½ tbsp. chopped Parsley

- 2 minced Sage leaves

- 1 tbsp. Olive Oil

- ¼ chopped onion (white)

- 1/16 tsp. Black Pepper (cracked)

- 1/2 tbsp. of Pepper Flakes (chili)

- ½ tsp. chopped rosemary

Directions:

1. Preheat oven to 400 degrees. Grease a baking sheet. Roast the squash in a preheated oven for 30 mins. Transfer it to a plate and let it cool. Sauté onion and garlic in the oil.

---

2. Now, scoop out the flesh from the roasted squash and add to the sautéed onion & garlic. Mash all of it well. Pour ½ quart of the broth into the slow cooker. Add the squash mixture. Cook on "low" for 4 hrs. Using a blender, make a smooth puree.

3. Transfer the puree to the slow cooker. Add in the rest of the broth and other ingredients. Cook again for 1 hr. on "high". Serve in heated soup bowls.

Nutrition:

Calories 158

Fats 6 g

Sodium 699 mg

Carbohydrates 24 mg

Fiber 6 g

Protein 3 g

Veggie and Beef Soup

Preparation time: 15 minutes

Cooking time: 4 hours

Servings: 4

Ingredients:

- 1 chopped Carrot

- 1 chopped Celery Rib

- ¾ l. Sirloin (ground)

- 1 cup Water

- ½ Butternut Squash (large)

- 1 clove Garlic

- ½ quart Beef broth

- 7 ounces diced Tomatoes (unsalted)

- ½ tsp. Kosher Salt

- 1 tbsp. chopped parsley

- ¼ tsp. Thyme (dried)

- ¼ tsp. Black Pepper (ground)

- ½ Bay Leaf

Directions:

1. Sauté all the vegetables in oil. Put the vegetables to the side, then place sirloin in the center. Sauté, using a spoon to crumble the meat. When cooked, combine with the vegetables on the sides of the pan.

2. Now, pour the rest of the ingredients into the slow cooker. Add cooked meat and vegetables. Stir well. Cook on "low" for 3 hrs. Serve in soup bowls.

Nutrition:

Calories 217

Fats 7 g

Cholesterol 53 mg

Sodium 728 mg

Carbohydrates 17 mg

Fiber 5 g

Protein 22 g

Collard, Sweet Potato and Pea Soup

Preparation time: 15 minutes

Cooking time: 4 hours

Servings: 4

Ingredients:

- 3 1/2 oz. Ham Steak, chopped

- ½ chopped Yellow Onion

- ½ lb. sliced Sweet Potatoes

- ¼ tsp. Red Pepper (hot and crushed)

- ½ cup frozen Peas (black-eyed)

- ½ tbsp. Canola Oil

- 1 minced clove of Garlic

- 1 ½ cup Water

- ¼ tsp. Salt

- 2 cups Collard Greens (julienned and without stems)

Directions:

1. Sauté ham with garlic and onion in oil. In a slow cooker, place other ingredients except for collard greens and peas.

2. Add in the ham mixture. Cook on "low" for 3 hrs. Now, add collard green and peas and cook again for an hour on "low." Serve in soup bowls.

Nutrition:

Calories 172

Fats 4 g

Sodium 547 mg

Carbohydrates 24 mg

Fiber 4 g

Protein 11 g

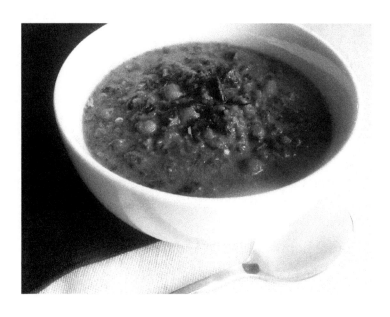

Bean Soup

Preparation time: 15 minutes

Cooking time: 5 hours

Servings: 4

Ingredients:

- ½ cup Pinto Beans (dried)

- ½ Bay Leaf

- 1 clove Garlic

- ½ onion (white)

- 2 cups Water

- 2 tbsp. Cilantro (chopped)

- 1 cubed Avocado

- 1/8 cup White Onion (chopped)

- ¼ cup Roma Tomatoes (chopped)

- 2 tbsp. Pepper Sauce (chipotle)

- ¼ tsp. Kosher Salt

- 2 tbsp. chopped Cilantro

- 2 tbsp. Low Fat Monterrey Jack Cheese, shredded

Directions:

1. Place water, salt, onion, pepper, garlic, bay leaf, and beans in the slow cooker. Cook on high for 5-6 hours. Discard the Bay leaf. Serve in heated bowls.

Nutrition:

Calories 258

Fats 19 g

Cholesterol 2 mg

Sodium 620 mg

Carbohydrates 25 mg

Fiber 11 g

Protein 8 g

Brown Rice and Chicken Soup

Preparation time: 15 minutes

Cooking time: 4 hours

Servings: 4

Ingredients:

- 1/3 cups Brown Rice

- 1 chopped Leek

- 1 sliced Celery Rib

- 1 ½ cups water

- ½ tsp. Kosher Salt

- ½ Bay Leaf

- 1/8 tsp. Thyme (dried)

- ¼ tsp. Black Pepper (ground)

- 1 tbsp. chopped parsley

- ½ quart Chicken Broth (low sodium)

- 1 sliced Carrot

- ¾ lb. of Chicken Thighs (skin and boneless)

Directions:

1. Boil 1 cup of water with ½ tsp. of salt in a saucepan. Add the rice. Cook for 30 mins on medium flame.

Brown chicken pieces in the oil. Transfer the chicken to a plate when done.

2. In the same pan, sauté the vegetables for 3 mins. Now, place the chicken pieces in the slow cooker. Add water and broth. Cook on "low" for 3 hrs. Put the rest of the fixing, the rice last. Cook again for 10 mins on "high." After discarding Bay leaf, serve in soup bowls

Nutrition:

Calories 208

Fats 6 g

Cholesterol 71 mg

Sodium 540 mg

Carbohydrates 18 mg

Fiber 2 g

Protein 20 g

Broccoli Soup

Preparation time: 15 minutes

Cooking time: 3 hours

Servings: 2

Ingredients:

- 4 cups chopped broccoli

- ½ cup chopped onion (white)

- 1 ½ cup Chicken Broth (low sodium)

- 1/8 tsp. Black Pepper (cracked)

- 1 tbsp. Olive Oil

- 1 Garlic Clove

- 1/16 tsp. Pepper Flakes (chili)

- ¼ cup Milk (low fat)

Directions:

1. In the slow cooker, cover the broccoli with water and cook for an hour on "high." Set aside after draining. Sauté onion and garlic in oil and transfer them to slow cooker when done. Add the broth.

2. Cook on "low" for 2 hrs. Transfer the mixture to a blender and make a smooth puree. Add black

pepper, milk, and pepper flakes to the puree. Boil briefly. Serve the soup in heated bowls.

Nutrition:

Calories 291

Fats 14 g

Cholesterol 24 mg

Sodium 227 mg

Carbohydrates 28 mg

Fiber 6 g

Protein 17 g

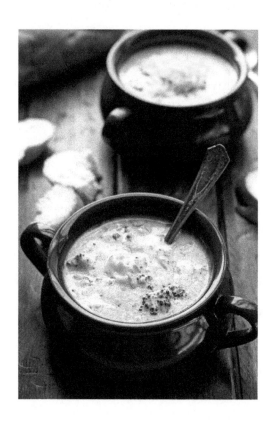

Hearty Ginger Soup

Preparation Time: 5 minutes

Cooking Time: 5 minutes

Servings: 4

Ingredients:

- 3 cups coconut almond milk

- 2 cups of water

- ½ pound boneless chicken breast halves, cut into chunks

- 3 tablespoons fresh ginger root, minced

- 2 tablespoons fish sauce

- ¼ cup fresh lime juice

- 2 tablespoons green onions, sliced

- 1 tablespoon fresh cilantro, chopped

Directions:

1. Take a saucepan and add coconut almond milk and water. Bring the mixture to a boil and add the chicken strips. Adjust the heat to medium, then simmer for 3 minutes. Stir in the ginger, lime juice, and fish sauce. Sprinkle a few green onions and cilantro.

Nutrition:

Calories: 415

Fat: 39g

Carbohydrates: 8g

Protein: 14g

Sodium: 150 mg

Tasty Tofu and Mushroom Soup

Preparation time: 15 minutes

Cooking time: 10 minutes

Servings: 8

Ingredients:

- 3 cups prepared dashi stock

- ¼ cup shiitake mushrooms, sliced

- 1 tablespoon miso paste

- 1 tablespoon coconut aminos

- 1/8 cup cubed soft tofu

- 1 green onion, diced

Directions:

1. Take a saucepan and add the stock; bring to a boil. Add mushrooms, cook for 4 minutes. Take a bowl and add coconut aminos, miso pastes, and mix well. Pour the mixture into stock and let it cook for 6 minutes on simmer. Add diced green onions and enjoy!

Nutrition:

Calories: 100

Fat: 4g

Carbohydrates: 5g

Protein: 11

Sodium: 87 mg

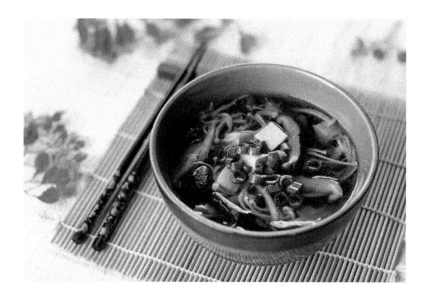

Ingenious Eggplant Soup

Preparation time: 15 minutes

Cooking time: 15 minutes

Servings: 8

Ingredients:

- 1 large eggplant, washed and cubed

- 1 tomato, seeded and chopped

- 1 small onion, diced

- 2 tablespoons parsley, chopped

- 2 tablespoons extra virgin olive oil

- 2 tablespoons distilled white vinegar

- ½ cup parmesan cheese, crumbled

- Sunflower seeds as needed

Directions:

1. Preheat your outdoor grill to medium-high. Pierce the eggplant a few times using a knife/fork. Cook the eggplants on your grill for about 15 minutes until they are charred. Put aside and allow them to cool.

2. Remove the eggplant's skin and dice the pulp. Put it in a mixing bowl and add parsley, onion, tomato,

olive oil, feta cheese, and vinegar. Mix well and chill for 1 hour. Season with sunflower seeds and enjoy!

Nutrition:

Calories: 99

Fat: 7g

Carbohydrates: 7g

Protein:3.4g

Sodium: 90 mg

Loving Cauliflower Soup

Preparation time: 15 minutes

Cooking time: 10 minutes

Servings: 6

Ingredients:

- 4 cups vegetable stock

- 1-pound cauliflower, trimmed and chopped

- 7 ounces Kite ricotta/cashew cheese

- 4 ounces almond butter

- Sunflower seeds and pepper to taste

Directions:

1. Put almond butter and melt in a skillet over medium heat. Add cauliflower and sauté for 2 minutes. Add stock and bring the mix to a boil.

2. Cook until cauliflower is al dente. Stir in cream cheese, sunflower seeds, and pepper. Puree the mix using an immersion blender. Serve and enjoy!

Nutrition:

Calories: 143

Fat: 16g

Carbohydrates: 6g

Protein: 3.4g

Sodium: 510 mg

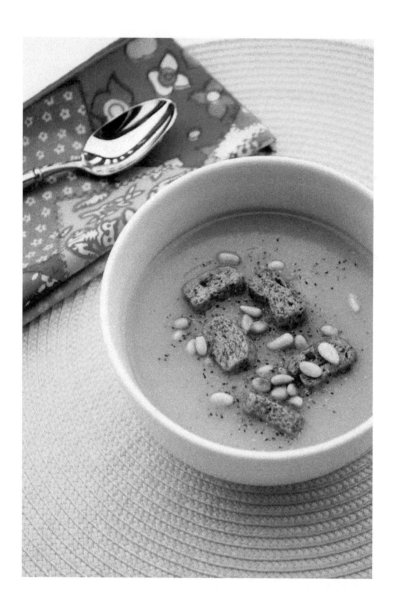

Garlic and Lemon Soup

Preparation time: 15 minutes

Cooking time: 0 minutes

Servings: 3

Ingredients:

- 1 avocado, pitted and chopped

- 1 cucumber, chopped

- 2 bunches spinach

- 1 ½ cups watermelon, chopped

- 1 bunch cilantro, roughly chopped

- Juice from 2 lemons

- ½ cup coconut aminos

- ½ cup lime juice

Directions:

1. Add cucumber, avocado to your blender, and pulse well. Add cilantro, spinach, and watermelon and blend. Add lemon, lime juice, and coconut amino. Pulse a few more times. Transfer to a soup bowl and enjoy!

Nutrition:

Calories: 100

Fat: 7g

Carbohydrates: 6g

Protein: 3g

Sodium: 0 mg

Cucumber Soup

Preparation time: 15 minutes

Cooking time: 0 minutes

Servings: 4

Ingredients:

- 2 tablespoons garlic, minced

- 4 cups English cucumbers, peeled and diced

- ½ cup onions, diced

- 1 tablespoon lemon juice

- 1 ½ cups vegetable broth

- ½ teaspoon sunflower seeds

- ¼ teaspoon red pepper flakes

- ¼ cup parsley, diced

- ½ cup Greek yogurt, plain

Directions:

1. Put the listed fixing in a blender and blend to emulsify (keep aside ½ cup of chopped cucumbers). Blend until smooth. Divide the soup amongst 4 servings and top with extra cucumbers. Enjoy chilled!

Nutrition:

Calories: 371

Fat: 36g

Carbohydrates: 8g

Protein: 4g

Sodium: 40 mg

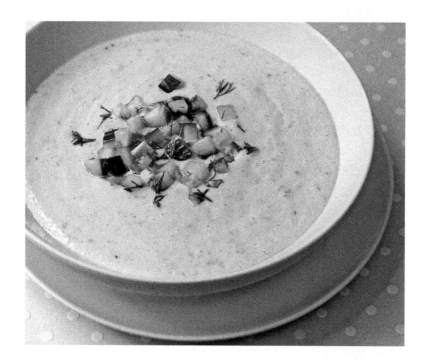

Roasted Garlic Soup

Preparation time: 15 minutes

Cooking time: 60 minutes

Servings: 10

Ingredients:

- 1 tablespoon olive oil

- 2 bulbs garlic, peeled

- 3 shallots, chopped

- 1 large head cauliflower, chopped

- 6 cups vegetable broth

- Sunflower seeds and pepper to taste

Directions:

1. Warm your oven to 400 degrees F. Slice ¼ inch top of the garlic bulb and place it in aluminum foil. Oiled it using olive oil and roast in the oven for 35 minutes. Squeeze flesh out of the roasted garlic.

2. Heat-up oil in a saucepan and add shallots, sauté for 6 minutes. Add garlic and remaining ingredients. Adjust heat to low. Let it cook for 15-20 minutes.

3. Puree the mixture using an immersion blender. Season soup with sunflower seeds and pepper. Serve and enjoy!

Nutrition:

Calories: 142

Fat: 8g

Carbohydrates: 3.4g

Protein: 4g

Sodium: 548 mg

Roasted Carrot Soup

Preparation time: 15 minutes

Cooking time: 50 minutes

Servings: 4

Ingredients:

- 8 large carrots, washed and peeled

- 6 tablespoons olive oil

- 1-quart broth

- Cayenne pepper to taste

- Sunflower seeds and pepper to taste

Directions:

1. Warm your oven to 425 degrees F. Take a baking sheet, add carrots, drizzle olive oil, and roast for 30-45 minutes. Put roasted carrots into a blender and add broth, puree. Pour into saucepan and heat soup. Season with sunflower seeds, pepper and cayenne. Drizzle olive oil. Serve and enjoy!

Nutrition:

Calories: 222

Fat: 18g

Net Carbohydrates: 7g

Protein: 5g

Sodium: 266 mg

Pumpkin Soup

Preparation time: 15 minutes

Cooking time: 6 hours

Servings: 4

Ingredients:

- 1 small pumpkin, halved, peeled, seeds removed, cubed

- 2 cups chicken broth

- 1 cup of coconut milk

- Pepper and thyme to taste

Directions:

1. Add all the ingredients to a crockpot. Cook for 6-8 hours on low. Make a smooth puree by using a blender. Garnish with roasted seeds. Serve and enjoy!

Nutrition:

Calories: 60

Fat: 2g

Carbohydrates: 10g

Protein: 3g

Sodium: 10 mg

Coconut Avocado Soup

Preparation time: 15 minutes

Cooking time: 10 minutes

Servings: 4

Ingredients:

- 2 cups vegetable stock

- 2 teaspoons Thai green curry paste

- Pepper as needed

- 1 avocado, chopped

- 1 tablespoon cilantro, chopped

- Lime wedges

- 1 cup of coconut milk

Directions:

1. Add milk, avocado, curry paste, pepper to a blender, and blend. Take a pan and place it over medium heat. Add mixture and heat, simmer for 5 minutes. Stir in seasoning, cilantro, and simmer for 1 minute. Serve and enjoy!

Nutrition:

Calories: 250

Fat: 30g

Carbohydrates: 2g

Protein: 4g

Sodium: 378 mg

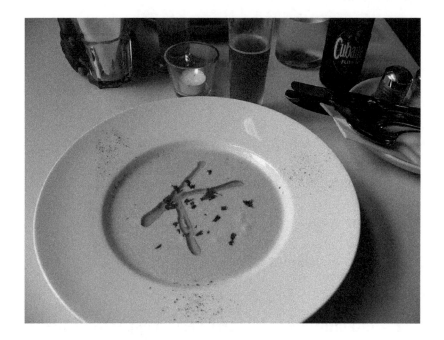

Coconut Arugula Soup

Preparation time: 15 minutes

Cooking time: 10 minutes

Servings: 4

Ingredients:

- Black pepper as needed

- 1 tablespoon olive oil

- 2 tablespoons chives, chopped

- 2 garlic cloves, minced

- 10 ounces baby arugula

- 2 tablespoons tarragon, chopped

- 4 tablespoons coconut milk yogurt

- 6 cups chicken stock

- 2 tablespoons mint, chopped

- 1 onion, chopped

- ½ cup of coconut milk

Directions:

1. Take a saucepan and place it over medium-high heat, add oil and let it heat up. Put onion and garlic and fry within 5 minutes. Stir in stock and reduce the heat, let it simmer.

2. Stir in tarragon, arugula, mint, parsley, and cook for 6 minutes. Mix in seasoning, chives, coconut yogurt, and serve.

Nutrition:

Calories: 180

Fat: 14g

Carbohydrates: 20g

Protein: 2g

Sodium: 362 mg

Cabbage Soup

Preparation time: 15 minutes

Cooking time: 25 minutes

Servings: 3

Ingredients:

- 3 cups non-fat beef stock

- 2 garlic cloves, minced

- 1 tablespoon tomato paste

- 2 cups cabbage, chopped

- ½ yellow onion

- ½ cup carrot, chopped

- ½ cup green beans

- ½ cup zucchini, chopped

- ½ teaspoon basil

- ½ teaspoon oregano

- Sunflower seeds and pepper as needed

Directions:

1. Grease a pot with non-stick cooking spray. Place it over medium heat and allow the oil to heat up. Add onions, carrots, and garlic, and sauté for 5 minutes.

Add broth, tomato paste, green beans, cabbage, basil, oregano, sunflower seeds, and pepper.

2. Boil the whole mix and reduce the heat, simmer for 5-10 minutes until all veggies are tender. Add zucchini and simmer for 5 minutes more. Sever hot and enjoy!

Nutrition:

Calories: 22

Fat: 0g

Carbohydrates: 5g

Protein: 1g

Sodium: 200 mg

Ginger Zucchini Avocado Soup

Preparation time: 15 minutes

Cooking time: 25 minutes

Servings: 3

Ingredients:

- 1 red bell pepper, chopped

- 1 big avocado

- 1 teaspoon ginger, grated

- Pepper as needed

- 2 tablespoons avocado oil

- 4 scallions, chopped

- 1 tablespoon lemon juice

- 29 ounces vegetable stock

- 1 garlic clove, minced

- 2 zucchinis, chopped

- 1 cup of water

Directions:

1. Take a pan and place over medium heat, add onion and fry for 3 minutes. Stir in ginger, garlic and cook for 1 minute. Mix in seasoning, zucchini stock, water, and boil for 10 minutes.

2. Remove soup from fire and let it sit; blend in avocado and blend using an immersion blender. Heat over low heat for a while. Adjust your seasoning and add lemon juice, bell pepper. Serve and enjoy!

Nutrition:

Calories: 155

Fat: 11g

Carbohydrates: 10g

Protein: 7g

Sodium: 345 mg

Greek Lemon and Chicken Soup

Preparation time: 15 minutes

Cooking time: 30 minutes

Servings: 4

Ingredients:

- 2 cups cooked chicken, chopped

- 2 medium carrots, chopped

- ½ cup onion, chopped

- ¼ cup lemon juice

- 1 clove garlic, minced

- 1 can cream of chicken soup, fat-free and low sodium

- 2 cans of chicken broth, fat-free

- ¼ teaspoon ground black pepper

- 2/3 cup long-grain rice

- 2 tablespoons parsley, snipped

Directions:

1. Put all of the listed fixings in a pot (except rice and parsley). Season with sunflower seeds and pepper. Bring the mix to a boil over medium-high heat. Stir in rice and set heat to medium.

2. Simmer within 20 minutes until rice is tender. Garnish parsley, and enjoy!

Nutrition:

Calories: 582

Fat: 33g

Carbohydrates: 35g

Protein: 32g

Sodium: 210 mg

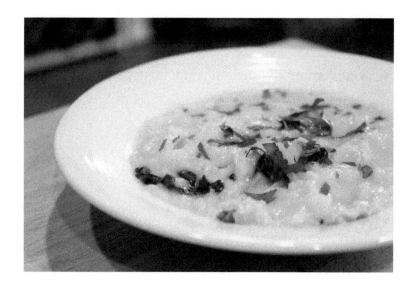

Garlic and Pumpkin Soup

Preparation time: 15 minutes

Cooking time: 5 hours

Servings: 4

Ingredients:

- 1-pound pumpkin chunks

- 1 onion, diced

- 2 cups vegetable stock

- 1 2/3 cups coconut cream

- ½ stick almond butter

- 1 teaspoon garlic, crushed

- 1 teaspoon ginger, crushed

- Pepper to taste

Directions:

1. Add all the fixing into your Slow Cooker. Cook for 4-6 hours on high. Puree the soup by using your immersion blender. Serve and enjoy!

Nutrition:

Calories: 235

Fat: 21g

Carbohydrates: 11g

Protein: 2g

Sodium: 395 mg

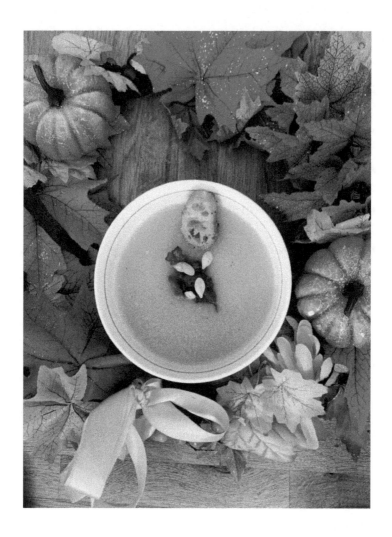

Golden Mushroom Soup

Preparation time: 15 minutes

Cooking time: 8 hours

Servings: 6

Ingredients:

- 1 onion, finely chopped

- 1 carrot, peeled and finely chopped

- 1 fennel bulb, finely chopped

- 1-pound fresh mushrooms, quartered

- 8 cups Vegetable Broth, Poultry Broth, or store-bought

- ¼ cup dry sherry

- 1 teaspoon dried thyme

- 1 teaspoon garlic powder

- ½ teaspoon of sea salt

- 1/8 teaspoon freshly ground black pepper

Directions:

1. In your slow cooker, combine all the ingredients, mixing to combine. Cover and set on low. Cook for 8 hours.

Nutrition:

Calories: 71

Fat: 0g

Carbohydrates: 15g

Fiber: 3g

Protein: 3g

Sodium: 650 mg

Minestrone

Preparation time: 15 minutes

Cooking time: 9 hours

Servings: 6

Ingredients:

- 2 carrots, peeled and sliced

- 2 celery stalks, sliced

- 1 onion, chopped

- 2 cups green beans, chopped

- 1 (16-ounce) can crushed tomatoes

- 2 cups cooked kidney beans, rinsed

- 6 cups Poultry Broth, Vegetable Broth, or store-bought

- 1 teaspoon garlic powder

- 1 teaspoon dried Italian seasoning

- ¼ teaspoon of sea salt

- ¼ teaspoon freshly ground black pepper

- 1½ cups cooked whole-wheat elbow macaroni (or pasta shape of your choice)

- 1 zucchini, chopped

Directions:

1. In your slow cooker, combine the carrots, celery, onion, green beans, tomatoes, kidney beans, broth, garlic powder, Italian seasoning, salt, and pepper in the slow cooker. Cook on low within 8 hours. Stir in the macaroni and zucchini. Cook on low within 1 hour more.

Nutrition:

Calories: 193

Fat: 0g

Carbohydrates: 39g

Fiber: 10g

Protein: 10g

Sodium: 100 mg

Butternut Squash Soup

Preparation time: 15 minutes

Cooking time: 8 hours

Servings: 6

Ingredients:

- 1 butternut squash, peeled, seeded, and diced

- 1 onion, chopped

- 1 sweet-tart apple (such as Braeburn), peeled, cored, and chopped

- 3 cups Vegetable Broth or store-bought

- 1 teaspoon garlic powder

- ½ teaspoon ground sage

- ¼ teaspoon of sea salt

- ¼ teaspoon freshly ground black pepper

- Pinch cayenne pepper

- Pinch nutmeg

- ½ cup fat-free half-and-half

Directions:

1. In your slow cooker, combine the squash, onion, apple, broth, garlic powder, sage, salt, black pepper, cayenne, and nutmeg. Cook on low within 8 hours.

2. Using an immersion blender, counter-top blender, or food processor, purée the soup, adding the half-and-half as you do. Stir to combine, and serve.

Nutrition:

Calories: 106

Fat: 0g

Carbohydrates: 26g

Fiber: 4g

Protein: 3g

Sodium: 550 mg

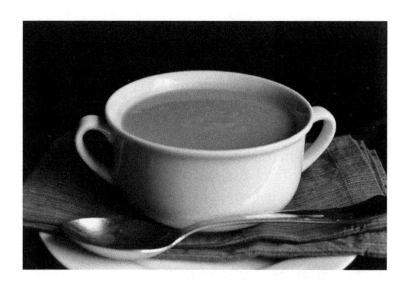

Black Bean Soup

Preparation time: 15 minutes

Cooking time: 8 hours

Servings: 6

Ingredients:

- 1-pound dried black beans, soaked overnight and rinsed

- 1 onion, chopped

- 1 carrot, peeled and chopped

- 2 jalapeño peppers, seeded and diced

- 6 cups Vegetable Broth or store-bought

- 1 teaspoon ground cumin

- 1 teaspoon ground coriander

- 1 teaspoon chili powder

- ½ teaspoon ground chipotle pepper

- ½ teaspoon of sea salt

- ¼ teaspoon freshly ground black pepper

- Pinch cayenne pepper

- ¼ cup fat-free sour cream, for garnish (optional)

- ¼ cup grated low-fat Cheddar cheese, for garnish (optional)

Directions:

1. In your slow cooker, combine all the fixing listed, then cook on low for 8 hours. If you'd like, mash the beans with a potato masher, or purée using an immersion blender, blender, or food processor. Serve topped with the optional garnishes, if desired.

Nutrition:

Calories: 320

Fat: 3g

Carbohydrates: 57g

Fiber: 13g

Protein: 18g

Sodium: 430 mg

Chickpea & Kale Soup

Preparation time: 15 minutes

Cooking time: 9 hours

Servings: 6

Ingredients:

- 1 summer squash, quartered lengthwise and sliced crosswise

- 1 zucchini, quartered lengthwise and sliced crosswise

- 2 cups cooked chickpeas, rinsed

- 1 cup uncooked quinoa

- 2 cans diced tomatoes, with their juice

- 5 cups Vegetable Broth, Poultry Broth, or store-bought

- 1 teaspoon garlic powder

- 1 teaspoon onion powder

- 1 teaspoon dried thyme

- ½ teaspoon of sea salt

- 2 cups chopped kale leaves

Directions:

1. In your slow cooker, combine the summer squash, zucchini, chickpeas, quinoa, tomatoes (with their juice), broth, garlic powder, onion powder, thyme, and salt. Cover and cook on low within 8 hours. Stir in the kale. Cover and cook on low for 1 more hour.

Nutrition:

Calories: 221

Fat: 3g

Carbohydrates: 40g

Fiber: 7g

Protein: 10g

Sodium: 124 mg

Clam Chowder

Preparation time: 15 minutes

Cooking time: 8 hours

Servings: 6

Ingredients:

- 1 red onion, chopped

- 3 carrots, peeled and chopped

- 1 fennel bulb and fronds, chopped

- 1 (10-ounce) can chopped clams, with their juice

- 1-pound baby red potatoes, quartered

- 4 cups Poultry Broth or store-bought

- ½ teaspoon of sea salt

- 1/8 teaspoon freshly ground black pepper

- 2 cups skim milk

- ¼ pound turkey bacon, browned and crumbled, for garnish

Directions:

1. In your slow cooker, combine the onion, carrots, fennel bulb and fronds, clams (with their juice), potatoes, broth, salt, and pepper. Cover and cook on

low within 8 hours. Stir in the milk and serve garnished with the crumbled bacon.

Nutrition:

Calories: 172

Fat: 1g

Carbohydrates: 29g

Fiber: 4g

Protein: 10g

Sodium: 517 mg

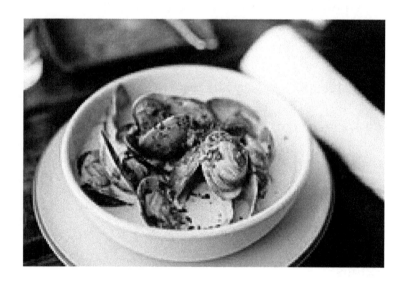

Chicken & Rice Soup

Preparation time: 15 minutes

Cooking time: 8 hours

Servings: 6

Ingredients:

- 1-pound boneless, skinless chicken thighs, cut into 1-inch pieces

- 1 onion, chopped

- 3 carrots, peeled and sliced

- 2 celery stalks, sliced

- 6 cups Poultry Broth or store-bought

- 1 teaspoon garlic powder

- 1 teaspoon dried rosemary

- ¼ teaspoon of sea salt

- ¼ teaspoon freshly ground black pepper

- 3 cups cooked Brown Rice

Directions:

1. In your slow cooker, combine the chicken, onion, carrots, celery, broth, garlic powder, rosemary, salt, and pepper. Cover and cook on low within 8 hours.

Stir in the rice about 10 minutes before serving, and allow the broth to warm it.

Nutrition:

Calories: 354

Fat: 7g

Carbohydrates: 43g

Fiber: 3g

Protein: 28g

Sodium: 610 mg

Tom Kha Gai

Preparation time: 15 minutes

Cooking time: 8 hours

Servings: 6

Ingredients:

- 1-pound boneless, skinless chicken thighs, cut into 1-inch pieces

- 1-pound fresh shiitake mushrooms halved

- 2 tablespoons grated fresh ginger

- 3 cups canned light coconut milk

- 3 cups Poultry Broth or store-bought

- 1 tablespoon Asian fish sauce

- 1 teaspoon garlic powder

- ¼ teaspoon freshly ground black pepper

- Juice of 1 lime

- 2 tablespoons chopped fresh cilantro

Directions:

1. In your slow cooker, combine the chicken thighs, mushrooms, ginger, coconut milk, broth, fish sauce, garlic powder, and pepper. Cover and cook on low

within 8 hours. Stir in the lime juice and cilantro just before serving.

Nutrition:

Calories: 481

Fat: 35g

Carbohydrates: 19g

Fiber: 5g

Protein: 28g

Sodium: 160 mg

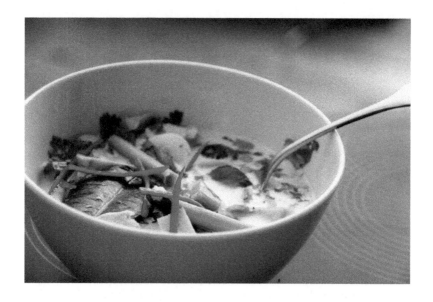

Chicken Corn Chowder

Preparation time: 15 minutes

Cooking time: 8 hours

Servings: 6

Ingredients:

- 1-pound boneless, skinless chicken thighs, cut into 1-inch pieces

- 2 onions, chopped

- 3 jalapeño peppers, seeded and minced

- 2 red bell peppers, seeded and chopped

- 1½ cups fresh or frozen corn

- 6 cups Poultry Broth or store-bought

- 1 teaspoon garlic powder

- ½ teaspoon of sea salt

- ¼ teaspoon freshly ground black pepper

- 1 cup skim milk

Directions:

1. In your slow cooker, combine the chicken, onions, jalapeños, red bell peppers, corn, broth, garlic powder, salt, and pepper. Cover and cook on low

within 8 hours. Stir in the skim milk just before serving.

Nutrition:

Calories: 236

Fat: 6g

Carbohydrates: 17g

Fiber: 3g

Protein: 27g

Sodium: 790 mg

Turkey Ginger Soup

Preparation time: 15 minutes

Cooking time: 8 hours

Servings: 6

Ingredients:

- 1-pound boneless, skinless turkey thighs, cut into 1-inch pieces

- 1-pound fresh shiitake mushrooms halved

- 3 carrots, peeled and sliced

- 2 cups frozen peas

- 1 tablespoon grated fresh ginger

- 6 cups Poultry Broth or store-bought

- 1 tablespoon low-sodium soy sauce

- 1 teaspoon toasted sesame oil

- 2 teaspoons garlic powder

- 1½ cups cooked Brown Rice

Directions:

1. In your slow cooker, combine the turkey, mushrooms, carrots, peas, ginger, broth, soy sauce, sesame oil, and garlic powder. Cover and cook on

low within 8 hours. About 30 minutes before serving, stir in the rice to warm it through.

Nutrition:

Calories: 318

Fat: 7g

Carbohydrates: 42g

Fiber: 6g

Protein: 24g

Sodium: 690 mg

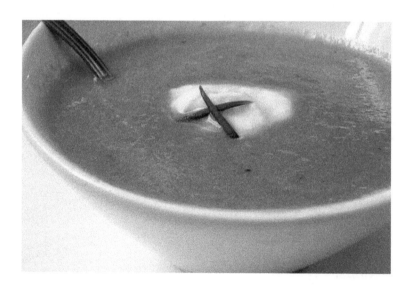

Italian Wedding Soup

Preparation time: 15 minutes

Cooking time: 7 hours

Servings: 6

Ingredients:

- 1-pound ground turkey breast

- 1½ cups cooked Brown Rice

- 1 onion, grated

- ¼ cup chopped fresh parsley

- 1 egg, beaten

- 1 teaspoon garlic powder

- 1 teaspoon sea salt, divided

- 6 cups Poultry Broth or store-bought

- 1/8 teaspoon freshly ground black pepper

- Pinch red pepper flakes

- 1-pound kale, tough stems removed, leaves chopped

Directions:

1. In a small bowl, combine the turkey breast, rice, onion, parsley, egg, garlic powder, and ½ teaspoon of sea salt. Roll the mixture into ½-inch meatballs and put them in the slow cooker.

2. Add the broth, black pepper, red pepper flakes, and the remaining ½ teaspoon of sea salt. Cover and cook on low for 7 to 8 hours. Before serving, stir in the kale. Cover and cook until the kale wilts.

Nutrition:

Calories: 302

Fat: 7g

Carbohydrates: 29g

Fiber: 3g

Protein: 29g

Sodium: 320 mg

Taco Soup

Preparation time: 15 minutes

Cooking time: 8 hours

Servings: 6

Ingredients:

- 1-pound ground turkey breast

- 1 onion, chopped

- 1 can tomatoes and green chilis, with their juice

- 6 cups Poultry Broth or store-bought

- 1 teaspoon chili powder

- 1 teaspoon ground cumin

- ½ teaspoon of sea salt

- ¼ cup chopped fresh cilantro

- Juice of 1 lime

- ½ cup grated low-fat Cheddar cheese

Directions:

1. Crumble the turkey into the slow cooker. Add the onion, tomatoes, green chilis (with their juice), broth, chili powder, cumin, and salt. Cover and cook on low within 8 hours. Stir in the cilantro and lime juice. Serve garnished with the cheese.

Nutrition:

Calories: 281

Fat: 10g

Carbohydrates: 20g

Fiber: 5g

Protein: 30g

Sodium: 470 mg

Italian Sausage & Fennel Soup

Preparation time: 15 minutes

Cooking time: 8 hours

Servings: 6

Ingredients:

- 1-pound Italian chicken or turkey sausage, cut into ½-inch slices

- 2 onions, chopped

- 1 fennel bulb, chopped

- 6 cups Poultry Broth or store-bought

- ¼ cup dry sherry

- 1½ teaspoons garlic powder

- 1 teaspoon dried thyme

- ½ teaspoon of sea salt

- ¼ teaspoon freshly ground black pepper

- Pinch red pepper flakes

Directions:

1. In your slow cooker, combine all the ingredients. Cover and cook on low within 8 hours.

Nutrition:

Calories: 311

Fat: 22g

Carbohydrates: 8g

Fiber: 2g

Protein: 18g

Sodium: 660 mg

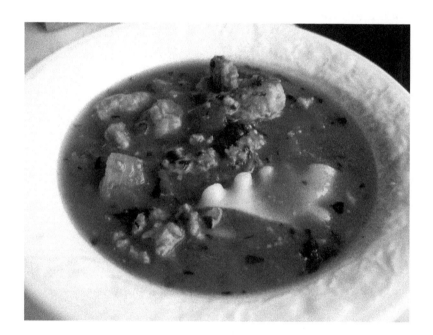

Beef & Barley Soup

Preparation time: 15 minutes

Cooking time: 8 hours

Servings: 6

Ingredients:

- 1-pound extra-lean ground beef

- 2 onions, chopped

- 3 carrots, peeled and sliced

- 1-pound fresh mushrooms, quartered

- 1½ cups dried barley

- 6 cups Beef Broth or store-bought

- 1 teaspoon ground mustard

- 1 teaspoon dried thyme

- 1 teaspoon garlic powder

- ¼ teaspoon of sea salt

- 1/8 teaspoon freshly ground black pepper

Directions:

1. In your slow cooker, crumble the ground beef into small pieces. Add the remaining ingredients. Cover and cook on low within 8 hours.

Nutrition:

Calories: 319

Fat: 5g

Carbohydrates: 44g

Fiber: 11g

Protein: 28g

Sodium: 380 mg

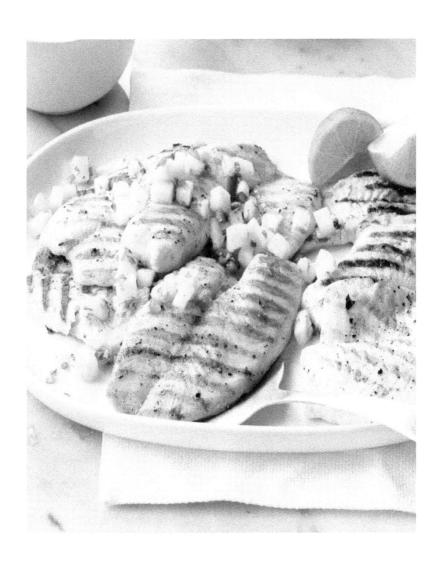

Lightning Source UK Ltd.
Milton Keynes UK
UKHW051223280321
380964UK00005B/41